STROKE AND DIABETES DIET COOKBOOK

Delicious Recipes for Stroke & Diabetes Management

T. John

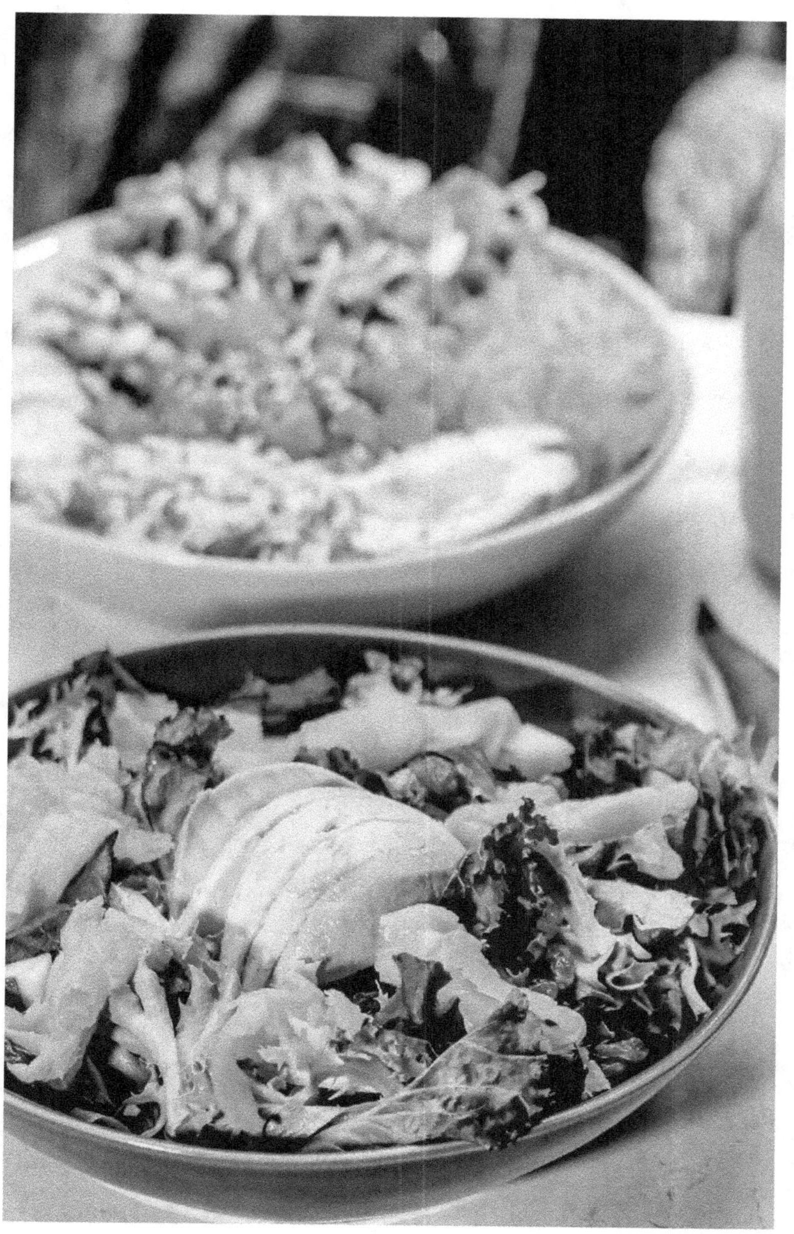

TABLE OF CONTENTS

Chapter 3: Lunch Recipes.. 48

Chapter 4: Dinner Recipes 71

Chapter 5: Snacks and Appetizers 95

INTRODUCTION

I magine your body's highways – the blood vessels. When you have diabetes, high blood sugar acts like rush hour traffic, constantly jamming the lanes. This can damage the vessel walls, making them more prone to blockages. Now, picture a stroke as a sudden road closure – a blood clot stopping vital oxygen and nutrients from reaching your brain. Scary, right?

Here's the good news: a healthy diet can be a powerful tool for managing both diabetes and stroke risk. It's like implementing traffic flow strategies to keep things moving smoothly. Let's delve deeper into this connection and how you can take charge of your health through mindful eating.

How Diabetes Increases Stroke Risk

Think of diabetes as a constant tug-of-war in your body. Your pancreas produces insulin, the key that unlocks your cells to absorb blood sugar. With diabetes, either the key isn't produced enough (Type 1) or the cells become resistant to it

(Type 2). This high blood sugar wreaks havoc on your blood vessels in two ways:

1. **Hardening of the Arteries (Atherosclerosis):** Over time, sugar sticks to the vessel walls, causing inflammation and the build-up of fatty deposits. This narrows the pathways, increasing the risk of clots that can trigger a stroke.
2. **Weakened Vessels:** High blood sugar can weaken the blood vessel walls themselves, making them more susceptible to rupturing and causing a stroke.

Diet as Your Traffic Control System

By adopting a stroke and diabetes-friendly diet, you can significantly improve blood sugar control and promote overall vascular health. Here are some key principles to follow:

- **Become Buddies with Fiber:** Fiber is like a traffic cop, regulating the flow of sugar into your bloodstream. Think whole grains, fruits (with skin!), and vegetables.

- **Lean Protein for Steady Energy:** Lean protein sources like fish, chicken, and legumes help you feel fuller for longer, preventing blood sugar spikes and crashes.

- **Healthy Fats are Your Friends:** Don't ditch all fats! Unsaturated fats from sources like olive oil, avocados, and nuts keep you satiated and improve blood vessel health.

- **Limit the Sugar Rush**: Added sugars and refined carbohydrates are like pouring gasoline on the blood sugar fire. Opt for natural sugars in fruits and limit sugary drinks, pastries, and white bread.

- **Portion Control is Key:** Even healthy foods can have consequences if overindulged. Use smaller plates, measure portions, and focus on mindful eating.

Tips for Success on Your Dietary Journey

- **Find a Support System**: Enlist a friend, family member, to be your cheerleader and guide.

- **Plan Your Meals:** Planning meals and snacks in advance prevents unhealthy choices when hunger strikes.

- **Spice Up Your Life!:** Explore new flavor combinations with herbs and spices. This keeps things interesting and reduces reliance on salt, which can elevate blood pressure.

- **Celebrate Non-Scale Victories**: Focus on how you feel – more energy, better sleep – rather than just the numbers on the scale.

- **Forgive Occasional Slip-Ups:** Don't beat yourself up for a misstep. Get back on track with the next meal.

Remember, a healthy diet for stroke and diabetes management is a lifestyle change, not a short-term fix. By making these adjustments and incorporating these tips, you're taking control of your health and paving the way for a brighter, healthier future.

Chapter 1: 30 Day Meal Plan

Week 1:

Day 1:

- Breakfast: Whole Grain Pancakes with Berries
- Lunch: Grilled Chicken Caesar Salad
- Dinner: Baked Salmon with Asparagus
- Snack: Greek Yogurt with Berries
- Dessert: Mixed Berry Crisp with Oat Topping

Day 2:

- Breakfast: Avocado and Egg Breakfast Wrap
- Lunch: Turkey and Veggie Wrap with Hummus
- Dinner: Lemon Herb Chicken with Roasted Vegetables
- Snack: Hummus and Veggie Sticks
- Dessert: Dark Chocolate Covered Strawberries

Day 3:

- Breakfast: Oatmeal with Fresh Fruit and Nuts

- Lunch: Quinoa and Black Bean Salad
- Dinner: Quinoa Stuffed Bell Peppers
- Snack: Cottage Cheese and Pineapple
- Dessert: Greek Yogurt Popsicles with Fruit

Day 4:

- Breakfast: Greek Yogurt Parfait with Granola
- Lunch: Tuna Salad Stuffed Bell Peppers
- Dinner: Shrimp and Broccoli Stir-Fry
- Snack: Trail Mix with Nuts and Dried Fruit
- Dessert: Baked Apples with Cinnamon

Day 5:

- Breakfast: Spinach and Feta Omelette
- Lunch: Mediterranean Chickpea Salad
- Dinner: Turkey Meatballs with Zucchini Noodles
- Snack: Whole Grain Crackers with Cheese
- Dessert: Chia Seed Pudding with Mango

Day 6:

- Breakfast: Quinoa Breakfast Bowl with Almonds and Berries
- Lunch: Salmon and Avocado Salad
- Dinner: Baked Cod with Lemon and Dill
- Snack: Edamame with Sea Salt
- Dessert: Banana Ice Cream with Almond Butter

Day 7:

- Breakfast: Veggie and Cheese Breakfast Casserole
- Lunch: Veggie and Brown Rice Sushi Rolls
- Dinner: Veggie Stir-Fry with Tofu
- Snack: Apple Slices with Almond Butter
- Dessert: Pumpkin Spice Muffins

Week 2:

Day 8:

- Breakfast: Breakfast Burrito with Black Beans and Salsa
- Lunch: Lentil Soup with Spinach
- Dinner: Grilled Steak with Cauliflower Mash

- Snack: Veggie Sushi Rolls
- Dessert: Avocado Chocolate Mousse

Day 9:

- Breakfast: Coconut Chia Pudding
- Lunch: Chicken and Veggie Stir-Fry
- Dinner: Eggplant Parmesan with Whole Wheat Pasta
- Snack: Deviled Eggs with Avocado
- Dessert: Lemon Blueberry Bars

Day 10:

- Breakfast: Banana Walnut Muffins
- Lunch: Stuffed Portobello Mushrooms
- Dinner: Thai Curry with Tofu and Vegetables
- Snack: Kale Chips with Parmesan
- Dessert: Coconut Macaroons

Day 11:

- Breakfast: Smoothie Bowl with Kale and Pineapple
- Lunch: Turkey Chili with Beans
- Dinner: Mediterranean Stuffed Chicken Breast

- Snack: Fruit Salad Skewers

- Dessert: Almond Flour Brownies

Day 12:

- Breakfast: Buckwheat Waffles with Apple Compote

- Lunch: Greek Salad with Grilled Shrimp

- Dinner: Beef and Vegetable Skewers

- Snack: Stuffed Mini Bell Peppers

- Dessert: Strawberry Frozen Yogurt Bark

Day 13:

- Breakfast: Veggie and Egg Breakfast Muffins

- Lunch: Caprese Salad with Balsamic Glaze

- Dinner: Ratatouille with Chickpeas

- Snack: Cucumber and Tomato Salad

- Dessert: Pineapple Sorbet

Day 14:

- Breakfast: Breakfast Quesadilla with Spinach and Cheese

- Lunch: Veggie and Hummus Sandwich

- Dinner: Spaghetti Squash with Tomato Sauce
- Snack: Roasted Chickpeas with Herbs
- Dessert: Carrot Cake Bites

Week 3:

Day 15:

- Breakfast: Whole Grain Pancakes with Berries
- Lunch: Minestrone Soup with Whole Wheat Pasta
- Dinner: Grilled Veggie Platter with Quinoa
- Snack: Hummus and Veggie Sticks
- Dessert: Berry Parfait with Greek Yogurt

Day 16:

- Breakfast: Avocado and Egg Breakfast Wrap
- Lunch: Grilled Chicken Caesar Salad
- Dinner: Baked Salmon with Asparagus
- Snack: Greek Yogurt with Berries
- Dessert: Mixed Berry Crisp with Oat Topping

Day 17:

- Breakfast: Oatmeal with Fresh Fruit and Nuts

- Lunch: Turkey and Veggie Wrap with Hummus
- Dinner: Lemon Herb Chicken with Roasted Vegetables
- Snack: Hummus and Veggie Sticks
- Dessert: Dark Chocolate Covered Strawberries

Day 18:

- Breakfast: Greek Yogurt Parfait with Granola
- Lunch: Quinoa and Black Bean Salad
- Dinner: Quinoa Stuffed Bell Peppers
- Snack: Cottage Cheese and Pineapple
- Dessert: Greek Yogurt Popsicles with Fruit

Day 19:

- Breakfast: Spinach and Feta Omelette
- Lunch: Tuna Salad Stuffed Bell Peppers
- Dinner: Shrimp and Broccoli Stir-Fry
- Snack: Trail Mix with Nuts and Dried Fruit
- Dessert: Baked Apples with Cinnamon

Day 20:

- Breakfast: Quinoa Breakfast Bowl with Almonds and Berries
- Lunch: Mediterranean Chickpea Salad
- Dinner: Turkey Meatballs with Zucchini Noodles
- Snack: Whole Grain Crackers with Cheese
- Dessert: Chia Seed Pudding with Mango

Day 21:

- Breakfast: Veggie and Cheese Breakfast Casserole
- Lunch: Salmon and Avocado Salad
- Dinner: Baked Cod with Lemon and Dill
- Snack: Edamame with Sea Salt
- Dessert: Banana Ice Cream with Almond Butter

Week 4:

Day 22:

- Breakfast: Breakfast Burrito with Black Beans and Salsa
- Lunch: Lentil Soup with Spinach
- Dinner: Grilled Steak with Cauliflower Mash

- Snack: Veggie Sushi Rolls
- Dessert: Avocado Chocolate Mousse

Day 23:

- Breakfast: Coconut Chia Pudding
- Lunch: Chicken and Veggie Stir-Fry
- Dinner: Eggplant Parmesan with Whole Wheat Pasta
- Snack: Deviled Eggs with Avocado
- Dessert: Lemon Blueberry Bars

Day 24:

- Breakfast: Banana Walnut Muffins
- Lunch: Stuffed Portobello Mushrooms
- Dinner: Thai Curry with Tofu and Vegetables
- Snack: Kale Chips with Parmesan
- Dessert: Coconut Macaroons

Day 25:

- Breakfast: Smoothie Bowl with Kale and Pineapple
- Lunch: Turkey Chili with Beans
- Dinner: Mediterranean Stuffed Chicken Breast

- Snack: Fruit Salad Skewers
- Dessert: Almond Flour Brownies

Day 26:

- Breakfast: Buckwheat Waffles with Apple Compote
- Lunch: Greek Salad with Grilled Shrimp
- Dinner: Beef and Vegetable Skewers
- Snack: Stuffed Mini Bell Peppers
- Dessert: Strawberry Frozen Yogurt Bark

Day 27:

- Breakfast: Veggie and Egg Breakfast Muffins
- Lunch: Caprese Salad with Balsamic Glaze
- Dinner: Ratatouille with Chickpeas
- Snack: Cucumber and Tomato Salad
- Dessert: Pineapple Sorbet

Day 28:

- Breakfast: Breakfast Quesadilla with Spinach and Cheese
- Lunch: Veggie and Hummus Sandwich

- Dinner: Spaghetti Squash with Tomato Sauce
- Snack: Roasted Chickpeas with Herbs
- Dessert: Carrot Cake Bites

Day 29:

- Breakfast: Whole Grain Pancakes with Berries
- Lunch: Minestrone Soup with Whole Wheat Pasta
- Dinner: Grilled Veggie Platter with Quinoa
- Snack: Hummus and Veggie Sticks
- Dessert: Berry Parfait with Greek Yogurt

Day 30:

- Breakfast: Avocado and Egg Breakfast Wrap
- Lunch: Grilled Chicken Caesar Salad
- Dinner: Baked Salmon with Asparagus
- Snack: Greek Yogurt with Berries
- Dessert: Mixed Berry Crisp with Oat Topping

Chapter 2: Breakfast Recipes

In this chapter, you'll find a variety of delicious breakfast recipes packed with wholesome ingredients to kickstart your mornings on the right note. From hearty pancakes to satisfying wraps and nourishing bowls, these recipes are designed to provide a balance of nutrients to fuel your day ahead.

Whole Grain Pancakes with Berries

Ingredients:

- 1 cup whole wheat flour
- 1 tablespoon baking powder
- 1 tablespoon honey
- 1 cup milk (or dairy-free alternative)
- 1 egg
- 1 teaspoon vanilla extract
- 1 cup mixed berries (strawberries, blueberries, raspberries)

Instructions:

1. In a mixing bowl, combine the whole wheat flour and baking powder.
2. In another bowl, whisk together the honey, milk, egg, and vanilla extract.
3. Pour the wet ingredients into the dry ingredients and stir until just combined.
4. Heat a non-stick skillet over medium heat and lightly grease with cooking spray.
5. Pour a quarter cup of batter onto the skillet for each pancake.
6. Cook until bubbles form on the surface, then flip and cook until golden brown.
7. Serve topped with mixed berries.

Nutrition Information (per serving):

- Calories: 250
- Protein: 8g
- Carbohydrates: 45g
- Fat: 4g
- Fiber: 6g
- Sugar: 12g
- Portion Size: 2 pancakes

Avocado and Egg Breakfast Wrap

Ingredients:

- 1 whole grain tortilla
- 1 ripe avocado, mashed
- 2 eggs, scrambled
- 1/4 cup diced tomatoes
- 2 tablespoons chopped cilantro
- Salt and pepper to taste

Instructions:

1. Warm the tortilla in a skillet or microwave.
2. Spread the mashed avocado evenly over the tortilla.
3. Top with scrambled eggs, diced tomatoes, and chopped cilantro.
4. Season with salt and pepper to taste.
5. Roll up the tortilla tightly and slice in half to serve.

Nutrition Information (per serving):

- Calories: 320
- Protein: 13g
- Carbohydrates: 22g

- Fat: 20g

- Fiber: 9g

- Sugar: 2g

- Portion Size: 1 wrap

Oatmeal with Fresh Fruit and Nuts

Ingredients:

- 1/2 cup rolled oats

- 1 cup water or milk (or dairy-free alternative)

- 1/2 cup fresh fruit (such as berries, sliced banana, or diced apple)

- 2 tablespoons chopped nuts (such as almonds, walnuts, or pecans)

- 1 tablespoon honey or maple syrup (optional)

Instructions:

1. In a saucepan, bring the water or milk to a boil.

2. Stir in the rolled oats and reduce heat to low.

3. Cook for 3-5 minutes, stirring occasionally, until oats are tender and creamy.

4. Remove from heat and transfer to a bowl.

5. Top with fresh fruit and chopped nuts.

6. Drizzle with honey or maple syrup if desired.

Nutrition Information (per serving):

- Calories: 300
- Protein: 8g
- Carbohydrates: 40g
- Fat: 12g
- Fiber: 6g
- Sugar: 12g
- Portion Size: 1 bowl

Greek Yogurt Parfait with Granola

Ingredients:

- 1/2 cup Greek yogurt
- 1/4 cup granola
- 1/4 cup mixed berries (such as strawberries, blueberries, raspberries)
- 1 tablespoon honey or maple syrup (optional)

Instructions:

1. In a glass or bowl, layer the Greek yogurt, granola, and mixed berries.
2. Repeat layers until ingredients are used up.
3. Drizzle with honey or maple syrup if desired.

Nutrition Information (per serving):

- Calories: 250
- Protein: 15g
- Carbohydrates: 30g
- Fat: 8g
- Fiber: 4g
- Sugar: 12g
- Portion Size: 1 parfait

Spinach and Feta Omelette

Ingredients:

- 2 eggs
- 1/4 cup baby spinach leaves
- 2 tablespoons crumbled feta cheese
- Salt and pepper to taste

- 1 teaspoon olive oil

Instructions:

1. In a bowl, beat the eggs until well combined.
2. Heat olive oil in a non-stick skillet over medium heat.
3. Pour the beaten eggs into the skillet.
4. Sprinkle spinach leaves and crumbled feta cheese evenly over the eggs.
5. Cook until the edges start to set, then carefully fold the omelette in half.
6. Cook for another minute until the eggs are fully cooked.
7. Season with salt and pepper to taste before serving.

Nutrition Information (per serving):

- Calories: 220
- Protein: 15g
- Carbohydrates: 2g
- Fat: 17g
- Fiber: 1g
- Sugar: 1g
- Portion Size: 1 omelette

Quinoa Breakfast Bowl with Almonds and Berries

Ingredients:

- 1/2 cup cooked quinoa
- 1/4 cup mixed berries (such as strawberries, blueberries, raspberries)
- 2 tablespoons sliced almonds
- 1 tablespoon honey or maple syrup (optional)

Instructions:

1. In a bowl, combine cooked quinoa, mixed berries, and sliced almonds.
2. Drizzle with honey or maple syrup if desired.
3. Stir to combine and serve immediately.

Nutrition Information (per serving):

- Calories: 280
- Protein: 9g
- Carbohydrates: 40g
- Fat: 9g
- Fiber: 6g

- Sugar: 12g
- Portion Size: 1 bowl

Veggie and Cheese Breakfast Casserole

Ingredients:

- 6 eggs
- 1 cup diced vegetables (such as bell peppers, onions, spinach)
- 1 cup shredded cheese (such as cheddar or mozzarella)
- Salt and pepper to taste
- Cooking spray

Instructions:

1. Preheat the oven to 350°F (175°C).
2. In a bowl, beat the eggs until well combined.
3. Stir in the diced vegetables and shredded cheese.
4. Season with salt and pepper to taste.
5. Grease a baking dish with cooking spray.
6. Pour the egg mixture into the baking dish.

7. Bake for 25-30 minutes, or until the eggs are set and the top is golden brown.

8. Allow the casserole to cool slightly before slicing and serving.

Nutrition Information (per serving):

- Calories: 220
- Protein: 15g
- Carbohydrates: 5g
- Fat: 15g
- Fiber: 1g
- Sugar: 2g
- Portion Size: 1 slice

Breakfast Burrito with Black Beans and Salsa

Ingredients:

- 1 whole grain tortilla
- 1/4 cup cooked black beans
- 2 tablespoons salsa
- 1 egg, scrambled

- 1/4 avocado, sliced

- Salt and pepper to taste

Instructions:

1. Warm the tortilla in a skillet or microwave.

2. Layer the black beans, salsa, scrambled egg, and sliced avocado on the tortilla.

3. Season with salt and pepper to taste.

4. Roll up the tortilla tightly and slice in half to serve.

Nutrition Information (per serving):

- Calories: 280

- Protein: 12g

- Carbohydrates: 30g

- Fat: 12g

- Fiber: 8g

- Sugar: 2g

- Portion Size: 1 burrito

Coconut Chia Pudding

Ingredients:

- 1/4 cup chia seeds
- 1 cup coconut milk (or dairy-free alternative)
- 1 tablespoon honey or maple syrup
- 1/4 teaspoon vanilla extract
- Sliced fruit for topping (such as mango, pineapple, or berries)

Instructions:

1. In a bowl, combine chia seeds, coconut milk, honey or maple syrup, and vanilla extract.
2. Stir well to mix all ingredients thoroughly.
3. Cover and refrigerate for at least 4 hours or overnight, until the mixture thickens and becomes pudding-like.
4. Stir the pudding before serving and top with sliced fruit.

Nutrition Information (per serving):

- Calories: 200

- Protein: 5g

- Carbohydrates: 20g

- Fat: 12g

- Fiber: 10g

- Sugar: 6g

- Portion Size: 1/2 cup

Banana Walnut Muffins

Ingredients:

- 1 cup whole wheat flour

- 1/2 cup oats

- 1 teaspoon baking powder

- 1/2 teaspoon baking soda

- 1/4 teaspoon salt

- 2 ripe bananas, mashed

- 1/4 cup honey or maple syrup

- 1/4 cup Greek yogurt

- 1 egg

- 1/4 cup chopped walnuts

Instructions:

1. Preheat the oven to 350°F (175°C).

2. In a bowl, combine whole wheat flour, oats, baking powder, baking soda, and salt.

3. In another bowl, mix mashed bananas, honey or maple syrup, Greek yogurt, and egg until well combined.

4. Gradually add the dry ingredients to the wet ingredients and stir until just combined.

5. Fold in the chopped walnuts.

6. Divide the batter evenly into muffin cups lined with paper liners.

7. Bake for 18-20 minutes, or until a toothpick inserted into the center comes out clean.

8. Allow the muffins to cool before serving.

Nutrition Information (per serving):

- Calories: 180
- Protein: 5g
- Carbohydrates: 30g
- Fat: 6g
- Fiber: 4g

- Sugar: 12g
- Portion Size: 1 muffin

Sweet Potato Hash with Turkey Sausage

Ingredients:

- 2 medium sweet potatoes, peeled and diced
- 1/2 lb turkey sausage, sliced
- 1 bell pepper, diced
- 1 small onion, diced
- 2 cloves garlic, minced
- 1 teaspoon paprika
- Salt and pepper to taste
- 1 tablespoon olive oil

Instructions:

1. Heat olive oil in a large skillet over medium heat.
2. Add the diced sweet potatoes and cook for 5-7 minutes, until slightly softened.
3. Add the turkey sausage, bell pepper, onion, and garlic to the skillet.

4. Season with paprika, salt, and pepper.

5. Cook, stirring occasionally, until sweet potatoes are tender and sausage is cooked through.

6. Serve hot, optionally garnished with chopped parsley or green onions.

Nutrition Information (per serving):

- Calories: 280
- Protein: 15g
- Carbohydrates: 25g
- Fat: 14g
- Fiber: 4g
- Sugar: 8g
- Portion Size: 1 cup

Smoothie Bowl with Kale and Pineapple

Ingredients:

- 1 cup frozen pineapple chunks
- 1/2 cup kale leaves, chopped
- 1/2 cup Greek yogurt

- 1/4 cup almond milk (or dairy-free alternative)
- 1 tablespoon honey or maple syrup (optional)
- Toppings: sliced banana, granola, shredded coconut, chia seeds

Instructions:

1. In a blender, combine frozen pineapple chunks, chopped kale, Greek yogurt, almond milk, and honey or maple syrup.
2. Blend until smooth and creamy, adding more almond milk if needed to reach desired consistency.
3. Pour the smoothie into a bowl.
4. Top with sliced banana, granola, shredded coconut, and chia seeds.
5. Serve immediately and enjoy with a spoon!

Nutrition Information (per serving):

- Calories: 250
- Protein: 10g
- Carbohydrates: 40g
- Fat: 6g
- Fiber: 8g

- Sugar: 28g
- Portion Size: 1 bowl

Buckwheat Waffles with Apple Compote

Ingredients:

- 1 cup buckwheat flour
- 1 teaspoon baking powder
- 1/2 teaspoon cinnamon
- 1 egg
- 1 cup almond milk (or dairy-free alternative)
- 2 tablespoons honey or maple syrup
- 1 teaspoon vanilla extract
- Cooking spray

For the Apple Compote:

- 2 apples, peeled and diced
- 2 tablespoons water
- 1 tablespoon honey or maple syrup
- 1/2 teaspoon cinnamon

Instructions:

1. In a large bowl, whisk together buckwheat flour, baking powder, and cinnamon.
2. In another bowl, beat the egg, then stir in almond milk, honey or maple syrup, and vanilla extract.
3. Pour the wet ingredients into the dry ingredients and mix until just combined.
4. Preheat a waffle iron and lightly coat with cooking spray.
5. Pour batter onto the waffle iron and cook according to manufacturer's instructions.
6. Meanwhile, prepare the apple compote by combining diced apples, water, honey or maple syrup, and cinnamon in a saucepan.
7. Cook over medium heat for 8-10 minutes, stirring occasionally, until apples are tender and mixture thickens.
8. Serve waffles topped with warm apple compote.

Nutrition Information (per serving):

- Calories: 280
- Protein: 7g

- Carbohydrates: 55g
- Fat: 5g
- Fiber: 7g
- Sugar: 25g
- Portion Size: 1 waffle with compote

Veggie and Egg Breakfast Muffins

Ingredients:

- 6 eggs
- 1/2 cup diced vegetables (such as bell peppers, onions, spinach)
- 1/4 cup shredded cheese (such as cheddar or mozzarella)
- Salt and pepper to taste
- Cooking spray

Instructions:

1. Preheat the oven to 350°F (175°C).
2. In a bowl, beat the eggs until well combined.
3. Stir in the diced vegetables and shredded cheese.
4. Season with salt and pepper to taste.

5. Grease a muffin tin with cooking spray.

6. Pour the egg mixture evenly into the muffin cups.

7. Bake for 20-25 minutes, or until the eggs are set and the tops are golden brown.

8. Allow the muffins to cool slightly before serving.

Nutrition Information (per serving):

- Calories: 150
- Protein: 10g
- Carbohydrates: 3g
- Fat: 10g
- Fiber: 1g
- Sugar: 1g
- Portion Size: 1 muffin

Breakfast Quesadilla with Spinach and Cheese

Ingredients:

- 2 whole grain tortillas
- 1 cup fresh spinach leaves

- 1/2 cup shredded cheese (such as cheddar or Monterey Jack)
- 2 eggs, scrambled
- Salsa or Greek yogurt for serving (optional)
- Cooking spray

Instructions:

1. Heat a skillet over medium heat and lightly coat with cooking spray.
2. Place one tortilla in the skillet and sprinkle half of the shredded cheese over it.
3. Layer spinach leaves and scrambled eggs on top of the cheese.
4. Sprinkle the remaining cheese over the eggs.
5. Top with the second tortilla.
6. Cook for 2-3 minutes on each side, until the tortillas are golden brown and the cheese is melted.
7. Remove from heat and let cool for a minute before slicing into wedges.
8. Serve with salsa or Greek yogurt if desired.

Nutrition Information (per serving):

- Calories: 320
- Protein: 18g
- Carbohydrates: 20g
- Fat: 18g
- Fiber: 3g
- Sugar: 2g
- Portion Size: 1 quesadilla

Chapter 3: Lunch Recipes

In this chapter, you'll find a selection of nutritious and delicious lunch recipes designed to keep you energized throughout the day. From satisfying salads to hearty soups and flavorful sandwiches, these recipes are packed with wholesome ingredients to support your health goals.

Grilled Chicken Caesar Salad

Ingredients:

- 2 boneless, skinless chicken breasts
- 1 head of romaine lettuce, chopped
- 1/4 cup grated Parmesan cheese
- 1/2 cup croutons
- Caesar dressing (store-bought or homemade)

Instructions:

1. Preheat grill to medium-high heat.
2. Season chicken breasts with salt and pepper.

3. Grill chicken for 6-8 minutes per side, or until cooked through.

4. Let chicken rest for 5 minutes, then slice into strips.

5. In a large bowl, toss chopped romaine lettuce with Caesar dressing.

6. Top with sliced grilled chicken, grated Parmesan cheese, and croutons.

7. Serve immediately.

Nutrition Information:

- Calories: 350
- Protein: 30g
- Carbohydrates: 15g
- Fat: 18g
- Fiber: 3g
- Sugar: 2g
- Portion Size: 1 serving

Turkey and Veggie Wrap with Hummus

Ingredients:

- 4 whole wheat tortillas
- 8 slices of turkey breast
- 1/2 cup hummus
- 1 cup mixed veggies (such as bell peppers, cucumber, and carrots), thinly sliced
- Handful of spinach leaves

Instructions:

1. Lay out tortillas and spread each with 2 tablespoons of hummus.
2. Layer each tortilla with 2 slices of turkey breast, mixed veggies, and spinach leaves.
3. Roll up tortillas tightly, folding in the sides as you go.
4. Slice wraps in half and serve.

Nutrition Information:

- Calories: 280

- Protein: 20g

- Carbohydrates: 30g

- Fat: 10g

- Fiber: 6g

- Sugar: 3g

- Portion Size: 1 wrap

Quinoa and Black Bean Salad

Ingredients:

- 1 cup cooked quinoa

- 1 can black beans, rinsed and drained

- 1 cup cherry tomatoes, halved

- 1/2 cup corn kernels (fresh or frozen)

- 1/4 cup red onion, finely chopped

- 1/4 cup fresh cilantro, chopped

- Juice of 1 lime

- Salt and pepper to taste

Instructions:

1. In a large bowl, combine cooked quinoa, black beans, cherry tomatoes, corn, red onion, and cilantro.

2. Drizzle lime juice over the salad and toss to combine.

3. Season with salt and pepper to taste.

4. Serve chilled or at room temperature.

Nutrition Information:

- Calories: 220
- Protein: 9g
- Carbohydrates: 40g
- Fat: 2g
- Fiber: 9g
- Sugar: 3g
- Portion Size: 1 cup

Tuna Salad Stuffed Bell Peppers

Ingredients:

- 2 cans of tuna, drained
- 1/4 cup Greek yogurt
- 1/4 cup diced celery
- 1/4 cup diced red onion
- 1/4 cup diced pickles
- Salt and pepper to taste

- 4 bell peppers, halved and seeds removed

Instructions:

1. In a mixing bowl, combine tuna, Greek yogurt, celery, red onion, and pickles.
2. Season with salt and pepper to taste and mix well.
3. Spoon tuna salad mixture into each bell pepper half.
4. Serve chilled or at room temperature.

Nutrition Information:

- Calories: 180
- Protein: 20g
- Carbohydrates: 10g
- Fat: 6g
- Fiber: 3g
- Sugar: 4g
- Portion Size: 1 stuffed bell pepper half

Mediterranean Chickpea Salad

Ingredients:

- 2 cups cooked chickpeas

- 1 cucumber, diced
- 1 cup cherry tomatoes, halved
- 1/4 cup red onion, finely chopped
- 1/4 cup Kalamata olives, sliced
- 1/4 cup crumbled feta cheese
- 2 tablespoons extra virgin olive oil
- 1 tablespoon red wine vinegar
- 1 teaspoon dried oregano
- Salt and pepper to taste

Instructions:

1. In a large bowl, combine chickpeas, cucumber, cherry tomatoes, red onion, olives, and feta cheese.
2. In a small bowl, whisk together olive oil, red wine vinegar, dried oregano, salt, and pepper.
3. Pour dressing over salad and toss to coat evenly.
4. Serve chilled or at room temperature.

Nutrition Information:

- Calories: 250
- Protein: 10g
- Carbohydrates: 25g

- Fat: 12g
- Fiber: 7g
- Sugar: 5g
- Portion Size: 1 cup

Salmon and Avocado Salad

Ingredients:

- 2 salmon fillets
- 4 cups mixed greens
- 1 avocado, sliced
- 1/4 cup cherry tomatoes, halved
- 1/4 cup sliced cucumber
- 1/4 cup sliced red onion
- 2 tablespoons balsamic vinaigrette
- Salt and pepper to taste

Instructions:

1. Preheat grill or oven to medium-high heat.
2. Season salmon fillets with salt and pepper.
3. Grill or bake salmon for 4-5 minutes per side, or until cooked through.

4. In a large bowl, toss mixed greens with balsamic vinaigrette.

5. Divide mixed greens among plates and top with sliced avocado, cherry tomatoes, cucumber, and red onion.

6. Place grilled salmon fillets on top of salads.

7. Serve immediately.

Nutrition Information:

- Calories: 380
- Protein: 25g
- Carbohydrates: 15g
- Fat: 25g
- Fiber: 7g
- Sugar: 5g
- Portion Size: 1 serving

Veggie and Brown Rice Sushi Rolls

Ingredients:

- 4 nori seaweed sheets
- 2 cups cooked brown rice

- 1 cucumber, julienned

- 1 carrot, julienned

- 1/2 avocado, sliced

- 1/4 cup pickled ginger

- 2 tablespoons low-sodium soy sauce

- Wasabi and/or sushi vinegar (optional)

Instructions:

1. Place a nori sheet on a sushi rolling mat or clean kitchen towel.

2. Spread a thin layer of brown rice evenly over the nori sheet, leaving a 1-inch border at the top.

3. Arrange cucumber, carrot, avocado, and pickled ginger in a line across the bottom third of the rice.

4. Starting from the bottom, roll the nori sheet tightly, using the sushi mat or towel to help.

5. Wet the top border of the nori sheet with water to seal the roll.

6. Slice the sushi roll into bite-sized pieces using a sharp knife.

7. Serve with low-sodium soy sauce, wasabi, and/or sushi vinegar if desired.

Nutrition Information:

- Calories: 220
- Protein: 6g
- Carbohydrates: 40g
- Fat: 4g
- Fiber: 7g
- Sugar: 2g
- Portion Size: 1 roll

Lentil Soup with Spinach

Ingredients:

- 1 cup dried lentils, rinsed
- 4 cups vegetable broth
- 1 onion, diced
- 2 carrots, diced
- 2 celery stalks, diced
- 2 cloves garlic, minced
- 1 teaspoon dried thyme
- 1 teaspoon dried oregano
- 2 cups fresh spinach leaves
- Salt and pepper to taste

Instructions:

1. In a large pot, combine lentils, vegetable broth, onion, carrots, celery, garlic, thyme, and oregano.
2. Bring to a boil over medium-high heat, then reduce heat to low and simmer for 20-25 minutes, or until lentils and vegetables are tender.
3. Stir in fresh spinach leaves and cook for an additional 2-3 minutes until wilted.
4. Season with salt and pepper to taste.
5. Serve hot.

Nutrition Information:

- Calories: 220
- Protein: 12g
- Carbohydrates: 40g
- Fat: 1g
- Fiber: 16g
- Sugar: 4g
- Portion Size: 1 cup

Chicken and Veggie Stir-Fry

Ingredients:

- 2 boneless, skinless chicken breasts, thinly sliced
- 2 cups mixed vegetables (such as bell peppers, broccoli, and snap peas), sliced
- 2 tablespoons low-sodium soy sauce
- 1 tablespoon sesame oil
- 2 cloves garlic, minced
- 1 teaspoon grated ginger
- Cooked brown rice or quinoa for serving

Instructions:

1. Heat sesame oil in a large skillet or wok over medium-high heat.
2. Add sliced chicken breast and cook until browned and cooked through, about 5-6 minutes.
3. Add mixed vegetables to the skillet and stir-fry for another 3-4 minutes, or until vegetables are tender-crisp.
4. Stir in minced garlic and grated ginger, and cook for an additional 1-2 minutes.

5. Drizzle low-sodium soy sauce over the stir-fry and toss to coat evenly.

6. Serve hot over cooked brown rice or quinoa.

Nutrition Information:

- Calories: 280
- Protein: 25g
- Carbohydrates: 20g
- Fat: 10g
- Fiber: 6g
- Sugar: 4g
- Portion Size: 1 serving

Stuffed Portobello Mushrooms

Ingredients:

- 4 large portobello mushrooms, stems removed
- 1 cup quinoa, cooked
- 1 cup spinach, chopped
- 1/2 cup cherry tomatoes, diced
- 1/4 cup feta cheese, crumbled
- 2 cloves garlic, minced

- 2 tablespoons olive oil
- Salt and pepper to taste

Instructions:

1. Preheat oven to 375°F (190°C).
2. In a large bowl, mix together cooked quinoa, chopped spinach, diced cherry tomatoes, crumbled feta cheese, minced garlic, olive oil, salt, and pepper.
3. Spoon quinoa mixture into the cavity of each portobello mushroom.
4. Place stuffed mushrooms on a baking sheet lined with parchment paper.
5. Bake in the preheated oven for 20-25 minutes, or until mushrooms are tender and filling is heated through.
6. Serve hot.

Nutrition Information:

- Calories: 220
- Protein: 10g
- Carbohydrates: 25g
- Fat: 10g

- Fiber: 5g

- Sugar: 3g

- Portion Size: 1 stuffed mushroom

Turkey Chili with Beans

Ingredients:

- 1 lb ground turkey

- 1 onion, diced

- 2 cloves garlic, minced

- 1 bell pepper, diced

- 1 can (14 oz) diced tomatoes

- 1 can (14 oz) kidney beans, rinsed and drained

- 1 can (14 oz) black beans, rinsed and drained

- 1 cup low-sodium chicken broth

- 2 tablespoons chili powder

- 1 teaspoon cumin

- Salt and pepper to taste

Instructions:

1. In a large pot, cook ground turkey over medium heat until browned.

2. Add diced onion, minced garlic, and diced bell pepper to the pot and cook for 3-4 minutes, until vegetables are softened.

3. Stir in diced tomatoes, kidney beans, black beans, chicken broth, chili powder, cumin, salt, and pepper.

4. Bring chili to a simmer and cook for 20-25 minutes, stirring occasionally.

5. Serve hot, garnished with your choice of toppings such as shredded cheese, chopped green onions, or Greek yogurt.

Nutrition Information:

- Calories: 300
- Protein: 25g
- Carbohydrates: 30g
- Fat: 10g
- Fiber: 10g
- Sugar: 5g
- Portion Size: 1 cup

Greek Salad with Grilled Shrimp

Ingredients:

- 1 lb shrimp, peeled and deveined
- 4 cups mixed greens
- 1 cucumber, sliced
- 1 cup cherry tomatoes, halved
- 1/4 cup sliced red onion
- 1/4 cup Kalamata olives
- 1/4 cup crumbled feta cheese
- 2 tablespoons extra virgin olive oil
- 1 tablespoon red wine vinegar
- 1 teaspoon dried oregano
- Salt and pepper to taste

Instructions:

1. Preheat grill to medium-high heat.
2. Thread shrimp onto skewers and season with salt, pepper, and a drizzle of olive oil.
3. Grill shrimp for 2-3 minutes per side, or until cooked through and slightly charred.

4. In a large bowl, toss mixed greens, cucumber, cherry tomatoes, red onion, Kalamata olives, and crumbled feta cheese.

5. In a small bowl, whisk together olive oil, red wine vinegar, dried oregano, salt, and pepper to make the dressing.

6. Drizzle dressing over salad and toss to coat evenly.

7. Top salad with grilled shrimp and serve immediately.

Nutrition Information:

- Calories: 280
- Protein: 25g
- Carbohydrates: 10g
- Fat: 15g
- Fiber: 3g
- Sugar: 5g
- Portion Size: 1 serving

Caprese Salad with Balsamic Glaze

Ingredients:

- 2 large tomatoes, sliced

- 1 ball fresh mozzarella cheese, sliced
- Fresh basil leaves
- Balsamic glaze
- Salt and pepper to taste

Instructions:

1. Arrange tomato and mozzarella slices on a serving platter, alternating and overlapping them.
2. Tuck fresh basil leaves between the tomato and mozzarella slices.
3. Drizzle balsamic glaze over the salad.
4. Season with salt and pepper to taste.
5. Serve immediately.

Nutrition Information:

- Calories: 200
- Protein: 12g
- Carbohydrates: 10g
- Fat: 12g
- Fiber: 3g
- Sugar: 5g
- Portion Size: 1 serving

Veggie and Hummus Sandwich

Ingredients:

- 4 slices whole grain bread
- 1/2 cup hummus
- 1 cucumber, thinly sliced
- 1 carrot, grated
- 1/4 cup alfalfa sprouts
- 1/4 cup baby spinach leaves
- Salt and pepper to taste

Instructions:

1. Spread hummus evenly on each slice of bread.
2. Layer cucumber slices, grated carrot, alfalfa sprouts, and baby spinach leaves on 2 slices of bread.
3. Season with salt and pepper to taste.
4. Top with the remaining slices of bread to form sandwiches.
5. Cut sandwiches in half and serve.

Nutrition Information:

- Calories: 280

- Protein: 10g

- Carbohydrates: 40g

- Fat: 10g

- Fiber: 8g

- Sugar: 5g

- Portion Size: 1 sandwich

Minestrone Soup with Whole Wheat Pasta

Ingredients:

- 4 cups low-sodium vegetable broth
- 1 can (14 oz) diced tomatoes
- 1 can (14 oz) kidney beans, rinsed and drained
- 1 cup chopped carrots
- 1 cup chopped celery
- 1 onion, diced
- 2 cloves garlic, minced
- 1 teaspoon dried basil
- 1 teaspoon dried oregano
- 1 cup whole wheat pasta
- Salt and pepper to taste

- Grated Parmesan cheese for serving (optional)

Instructions:

1. In a large pot, combine vegetable broth, diced tomatoes, kidney beans, chopped carrots, chopped celery, diced onion, minced garlic, dried basil, and dried oregano.
2. Bring to a boil over medium-high heat, then reduce heat to low and simmer for 15-20 minutes.
3. Add whole wheat pasta to the pot and cook according to package instructions, until pasta is tender.
4. Season with salt and pepper to taste.
5. Serve hot, garnished with grated Parmesan cheese if desired.

Nutrition Information:

- Calories: 250
- Protein: 10g
- Carbohydrates: 45g
- Fat: 3g
- Fiber: 10g
- Sugar: 8g
- Portion Size: 1 cup

Chapter 4: Dinner Recipes

These recipes are carefully crafted with wholesome ingredients and simple instructions to make your evenings both nutritious and enjoyable. From succulent seafood to hearty vegetarian options, there's something here for everyone. Let's dive in!

Baked Salmon with Asparagus

Ingredients:

- 4 salmon fillets
- 1 bunch of asparagus
- Olive oil
- Lemon slices
- Salt and pepper

Instructions:

1. Preheat oven to 400°F (200°C).
2. Place salmon fillets on a baking sheet lined with parchment paper.

3. Arrange asparagus spears around the salmon.

4. Drizzle with olive oil and season with salt and pepper.

5. Place lemon slices on top of the salmon.

6. Bake for 12-15 minutes, or until salmon is cooked through.

7. Serve hot.

Nutrition Information:

- Calories: 300
- Protein: 25g
- Carbohydrates: 5g
- Fat: 18g
- Fiber: 2g
- Sugar: 2g
- Portion Size: 1 fillet with asparagus

Lemon Herb Chicken with Roasted Vegetables

Ingredients:

- 4 chicken breasts

- Assorted vegetables (such as carrots, bell peppers, and potatoes)
- Olive oil
- Lemon juice
- Garlic
- Mixed herbs (such as rosemary, thyme, and oregano)
- Salt and pepper

Instructions:

1. Preheat oven to 375°F (190°C).
2. Place chicken breasts and chopped vegetables on a baking sheet.
3. Drizzle with olive oil and lemon juice.
4. Season with minced garlic, mixed herbs, salt, and pepper.
5. Roast for 25-30 minutes, or until chicken is cooked through and vegetables are tender.
6. Serve hot.

Nutrition Information:

- Calories: 350
- Protein: 30g

- Carbohydrates: 15g

- Fat: 15g

- Fiber: 5g

- Sugar: 5g

- Portion Size: 1 chicken breast with vegetables

Quinoa Stuffed Bell Peppers

Ingredients:

- 4 bell peppers

- 1 cup quinoa, cooked

- 1 can black beans, drained and rinsed

- 1 cup corn kernels

- 1 cup diced tomatoes

- 1 teaspoon chili powder

- 1/2 teaspoon cumin

- Salt and pepper

- Shredded cheese (optional)

Instructions:

1. Preheat oven to 375°F (190°C).

2. Cut the tops off the bell peppers and remove the seeds and membranes.

3. In a bowl, mix cooked quinoa, black beans, corn, diced tomatoes, chili powder, cumin, salt, and pepper.

4. Stuff the bell peppers with the quinoa mixture.

5. Place the stuffed peppers in a baking dish and cover with foil.

6. Bake for 25-30 minutes, or until peppers are tender.

7. Optionally, sprinkle shredded cheese on top and bake for an additional 5 minutes until melted.

8. Serve hot.

Nutrition Information:
- Calories: 300
- Protein: 12g
- Carbohydrates: 50g
- Fat: 5g
- Fiber: 10g
- Sugar: 8g
- Portion Size: 1 stuffed pepper

Shrimp and Broccoli Stir-Fry

Ingredients:

- 1 lb shrimp, peeled and deveined
- 2 cups broccoli florets
- 1 bell pepper, sliced
- 1 onion, sliced
- 2 cloves garlic, minced
- Soy sauce
- Sesame oil
- Red pepper flakes (optional)
- Cooked rice, for serving

Instructions:

1. Heat sesame oil in a large skillet over medium heat.
2. Add minced garlic and cook until fragrant.
3. Add shrimp to the skillet and cook until pink.
4. Stir in broccoli florets, sliced bell pepper, and onion.
5. Drizzle with soy sauce and cook until vegetables are tender-crisp.
6. Sprinkle with red pepper flakes if desired.
7. Serve over cooked rice.

Nutrition Information:

- Calories: 250
- Protein: 25g
- Carbohydrates: 15g
- Fat: 8g
- Fiber: 5g
- Sugar: 5g
- Portion Size: 1 cup of stir-fry with rice

Turkey Meatballs with Zucchini Noodles

Ingredients:

- 1 lb ground turkey
- 1 egg
- 1/4 cup breadcrumbs
- 2 cloves garlic, minced
- 1 teaspoon Italian seasoning
- Salt and pepper
- 4 medium zucchinis
- Olive oil
- Marinara sauce

Instructions:

1. In a bowl, mix ground turkey, egg, breadcrumbs, minced garlic, Italian seasoning, salt, and pepper.
2. Form the mixture into meatballs.
3. Heat olive oil in a skillet over medium heat.
4. Add the meatballs to the skillet and cook until browned on all sides and cooked through.
5. Spiralize the zucchinis to create noodles.
6. In the same skillet, add the zucchini noodles and cook until tender.
7. Serve the turkey meatballs over the zucchini noodles with marinara sauce.

Nutrition Information:

- Calories: 300
- Protein: 25g
- Carbohydrates: 10g
- Fat: 15g
- Fiber: 3g
- Sugar: 5g
- Portion Size: 3-4 meatballs with zucchini noodles

Baked Cod with Lemon and Dill

Ingredients:

- 4 cod fillets
- Lemon slices
- Fresh dill
- Olive oil
- Salt and pepper

Instructions:

1. Preheat oven to 400°F (200°C).
2. Place cod fillets on a baking sheet lined with parchment paper.
3. Drizzle with olive oil and season with salt and pepper.
4. Place lemon slices on top of the cod fillets.
5. Sprinkle with fresh dill.
6. Bake for 12-15 minutes, or until cod is cooked through and flakes easily with a fork.
7. Serve hot.

Nutrition Information:

- Calories: 200
- Protein: 30g
- Carbohydrates: 1g
- Fat: 8g
- Fiber: 0g
- Sugar: 0g
- Portion Size: 1 cod fillet with lemon and dill

Veggie Stir-Fry with Tofu

Ingredients:

- 1 block tofu, pressed and cubed
- Assorted vegetables (such as bell peppers, broccoli, carrots, and snap peas)
- Soy sauce
- Sesame oil
- Garlic powder
- Ginger powder
- Red pepper flakes (optional)
- Cooked rice, for serving

Instructions:

1. Heat sesame oil in a large skillet or wok over medium-high heat.
2. Add cubed tofu to the skillet and cook until browned on all sides.
3. Add assorted vegetables to the skillet and stir-fry until tender-crisp.
4. Season with soy sauce, garlic powder, ginger powder, and red pepper flakes if desired.
5. Continue to stir-fry until everything is well combined and heated through.
6. Serve over cooked rice.

Nutrition Information:
- Calories: 250
- Protein: 15g
- Carbohydrates: 20g
- Fat: 10g
- Fiber: 5g
- Sugar: 5g
- Portion Size: 1 cup of stir-fry with rice

Grilled Steak with Cauliflower Mash

Ingredients:

- 4 steak cuts (such as sirloin or ribeye)
- Salt and pepper
- Olive oil
- 1 head cauliflower, chopped into florets
- Garlic cloves, minced
- Butter
- Milk (optional)
- Chives, chopped (optional)

Instructions:

1. Preheat grill to medium-high heat.
2. Season steak cuts with salt, pepper, and olive oil.
3. Grill steaks for 4-5 minutes on each side for medium-rare (adjust cooking time according to desired doneness).
4. Meanwhile, steam cauliflower florets until tender.
5. In a blender or food processor, blend steamed cauliflower with minced garlic, butter, and milk (if using) until smooth.
6. Season with salt and pepper to taste.

7. Serve grilled steak with cauliflower mash.

8. Garnish with chopped chives if desired.

Nutrition Information:

- Calories: 400

- Protein: 40g

- Carbohydrates: 10g

- Fat: 20g

- Fiber: 5g

- Sugar: 5g

- Portion Size: 1 steak with cauliflower mash

Eggplant Parmesan with Whole Wheat Pasta

Ingredients:

- 1 large eggplant, sliced into rounds

- Whole wheat pasta

- Marinara sauce

- Mozzarella cheese, shredded

- Parmesan cheese, grated

- Fresh basil leaves

- Olive oil

- Salt and pepper

Instructions:

1. Preheat oven to 375°F (190°C).

2. Arrange eggplant slices on a baking sheet lined with parchment paper.

3. Drizzle with olive oil and season with salt and pepper.

4. Bake for 20-25 minutes, or until eggplant is tender and lightly browned.

5. Cook whole wheat pasta according to package instructions.

6. In a baking dish, layer cooked pasta, marinara sauce, baked eggplant slices, and shredded mozzarella cheese.

7. Repeat the layers until all ingredients are used, ending with a layer of cheese on top.

8. Sprinkle grated Parmesan cheese over the top.

9. Bake for 25-30 minutes, or until cheese is melted and bubbly.

10. Garnish with fresh basil leaves before serving.

Nutrition Information:

- Calories: 350
- Protein: 15g
- Carbohydrates: 45g
- Fat: 12g
- Fiber: 8g
- Sugar: 10g
- Portion Size: 1 cup of eggplant parmesan with pasta

Thai Curry with Tofu and Vegetables

Ingredients:

- 1 block tofu, pressed and cubed
- Assorted vegetables (such as bell peppers, carrots, zucchini, and snow peas)
- Thai curry paste
- Coconut milk
- Soy sauce
- Brown sugar
- Lime juice
- Fresh cilantro leaves
- Cooked rice, for serving

Instructions:

1. Heat coconut milk in a large skillet or wok over medium heat.
2. Add Thai curry paste to the skillet and stir until fragrant.
3. Stir in cubed tofu and assorted vegetables.
4. Season with soy sauce, brown sugar, and lime juice.
5. Simmer for 10-15 minutes, or until vegetables are tender and tofu is heated through.
6. Serve over cooked rice.
7. Garnish with fresh cilantro leaves before serving.

Nutrition Information:

- Calories: 300
- Protein: 15g
- Carbohydrates: 30g
- Fat: 15g
- Fiber: 8g
- Sugar: 10g
- Portion Size: 1 cup of curry with rice

Mediterranean Stuffed Chicken Breast

Ingredients:

- 4 boneless, skinless chicken breasts
- Spinach leaves
- Sun-dried tomatoes, chopped
- Kalamata olives, chopped
- Feta cheese, crumbled
- Olive oil
- Garlic powder
- Dried oregano
- Salt and pepper

Instructions:

1. Preheat oven to 375°F (190°C).
2. Butterfly each chicken breast by slicing horizontally through the middle, but not all the way through.
3. Open each chicken breast and season the inside with garlic powder, dried oregano, salt, and pepper.
4. Layer spinach leaves, sun-dried tomatoes, chopped olives, and crumbled feta cheese on one side of each chicken breast.

5. Fold the other side of the chicken breast over the filling to close.

6. Secure with toothpicks if necessary.

7. Heat olive oil in an oven-safe skillet over medium-high heat.

8. Sear stuffed chicken breasts for 2-3 minutes on each side until browned.

9. Transfer the skillet to the oven and bake for 20-25 minutes, or until chicken is cooked through.

10. Serve hot.

Nutrition Information:

- Calories: 350
- Protein: 40g
- Carbohydrates: 5g
- Fat: 18g
- Fiber: 2g
- Sugar: 2g
- Portion Size: 1 stuffed chicken breast

Beef and Vegetable Skewers

Ingredients:

- 1 lb beef sirloin, cubed
- Assorted vegetables (such as bell peppers, onions, mushrooms, and cherry tomatoes)
- Olive oil
- Garlic powder
- Dried thyme
- Salt and pepper

Instructions:

1. Preheat grill to medium-high heat.
2. Thread beef cubes and assorted vegetables onto skewers.
3. Drizzle skewers with olive oil and season with garlic powder, dried thyme, salt, and pepper.
4. Grill skewers for 10-12 minutes, turning occasionally, until beef is cooked to desired doneness and vegetables are tender.
5. Serve hot.

Nutrition Information:

- Calories: 300
- Protein: 30g
- Carbohydrates: 10g
- Fat: 15g
- Fiber: 3g
- Sugar: 5g
- Portion Size: 1 skewer with vegetables

Ratatouille with Chickpeas

Ingredients:

- 1 eggplant, diced
- 2 zucchinis, diced
- 1 bell pepper, diced
- 1 onion, diced
- 2 cloves garlic, minced
- 1 can chickpeas, drained and rinsed
- 1 can diced tomatoes
- Olive oil
- Herbes de Provence
- Salt and pepper

Instructions:

1. Heat olive oil in a large skillet or pot over medium heat.
2. Add diced onion and minced garlic, and cook until softened.
3. Add diced eggplant, zucchinis, and bell pepper to the skillet.
4. Cook until vegetables are tender.
5. Stir in drained and rinsed chickpeas and diced tomatoes.
6. Season with herbes de Provence, salt, and pepper.
7. Simmer for 10-15 minutes to allow flavors to meld.
8. Serve hot.

Nutrition Information:

- Calories: 250
- Protein: 10g
- Carbohydrates: 40g
- Fat: 8g
- Fiber: 12g
- Sugar: 10g
- Portion Size: 1 cup of ratatouille

Spaghetti Squash with Tomato Sauce

Ingredients:

- 1 spaghetti squash
- Marinara sauce
- Fresh basil leaves
- Parmesan cheese, grated
- Olive oil
- Salt and pepper

Instructions:

1. Preheat oven to 400°F (200°C).
2. Cut spaghetti squash in half lengthwise and scoop out the seeds.
3. Drizzle with olive oil and season with salt and pepper.
4. Place spaghetti squash halves cut-side down on a baking sheet lined with parchment paper.
5. Bake for 30-40 minutes, or until squash is tender and can be easily pierced with a fork.
6. Use a fork to scrape the flesh of the spaghetti squash into strands.

7. Serve with marinara sauce.

8. Garnish with fresh basil leaves and grated Parmesan cheese.

Nutrition Information:

- Calories: 200
- Protein: 5g
- Carbohydrates: 30g
- Fat: 8g
- Fiber: 8g
- Sugar: 10g
- Portion Size: 1 cup of spaghetti squash with sauce

Grilled Veggie Platter with Quinoa

Ingredients:

- Assorted vegetables (such as bell peppers, zucchini, mushrooms, and cherry tomatoes)
- Cooked quinoa
- Balsamic vinegar
- Olive oil
- Garlic powder

- Italian seasoning
- Salt and pepper

Instructions:

1. Preheat grill to medium-high heat.

2. Toss assorted vegetables with olive oil, balsamic vinegar, garlic powder, Italian seasoning, salt, and pepper.

3. Grill vegetables for 8-10 minutes, turning occasionally, until tender and slightly charred.

4. Serve grilled vegetables with cooked quinoa.

5. Drizzle with additional balsamic vinegar if desired.

Nutrition Information:

- Calories: 250
- Protein: 8g
- Carbohydrates: 40g
- Fat: 5g
- Fiber: 10g
- Sugar: 8g
- Portion Size: 1 cup of grilled vegetables with quinoa

Chapter 5: Snacks and Appetizers

In this chapter, we've curated a selection of snacks and appetizers designed to tantalize your taste buds while keeping you on track with your health goals. From crunchy veggies with creamy dips to protein-packed bites and fruity delights, these recipes offer a balance of flavors and nutrients to support your well-being.

Hummus and Veggie Sticks

Ingredients:

- 1 cup hummus
- Assorted vegetables (carrots, celery, bell peppers, cucumber)

Instructions:

1. Wash and cut the vegetables into sticks.
2. Serve with hummus for dipping.

Nutrition Information:

- Calories: 150
- Protein: 6g
- Carbohydrates: 20g
- Fat: 6g
- Fiber: 8g
- Sugar: 3g
- Portion Size: 1/2 cup hummus and 1 cup vegetables

Guacamole with Baked Tortilla Chips

Ingredients:

- 2 ripe avocados
- 1 tomato, diced
- 1/4 cup red onion, finely chopped
- 1/4 cup cilantro, chopped
- Juice of 1 lime
- Salt and pepper to taste
- Whole grain tortilla chips

Instructions:

1. In a bowl, mash the avocados with a fork.

2. Add diced tomato, red onion, cilantro, lime juice, salt, and pepper. Mix well.

3. Serve with baked tortilla chips.

Nutrition Information:

- Calories: 180
- Protein: 4g
- Carbohydrates: 15g
- Fat: 12g
- Fiber: 8g
- Sugar: 2g
- Portion Size: 1/4 cup guacamole and 10 tortilla chips

Greek Yogurt with Berries

Ingredients:

- 1 cup Greek yogurt
- Assorted berries (strawberries, blueberries, raspberries)

Instructions:

1. Spoon Greek yogurt into a bowl.

2. Top with fresh berries.

3. Enjoy immediately.

Nutrition Information:

- Calories: 120

- Protein: 15g

- Carbohydrates: 10g

- Fat: 2g

- Fiber: 2g

- Sugar: 8g

- Portion Size: 1 cup yogurt and 1/2 cup berries

Cottage Cheese and Pineapple

Ingredients:

- 1/2 cup cottage cheese

- 1/2 cup pineapple chunks (fresh or canned in juice)

Instructions:

1. Place cottage cheese in a bowl.

2. Top with pineapple chunks.

3. Serve chilled.

Nutrition Information:

- Calories: 120

- Protein: 13g

- Carbohydrates: 15g

- Fat: 2g

- Fiber: 1g

- Sugar: 12g

- Portion Size: 1/2 cup cottage cheese and 1/2 cup pineapple

Trail Mix with Nuts and Dried Fruit

Ingredients:

- 1/4 cup almonds

- 1/4 cup cashews

- 1/4 cup dried cranberries

- 1/4 cup raisins

Instructions:

1. Mix all ingredients together in a bowl.

2. Portion into small snack bags for easy grab-and-go.

Nutrition Information:

*   Calories: 200

*   Protein: 6g

*   Carbohydrates: 20g

*   Fat: 12g

*   Fiber: 4g

*   Sugar: 12g

*   Portion Size: 1/4 cup trail mix

Whole Grain Crackers with Cheese

Ingredients:

*   Whole grain crackers

*   Slices of cheese (cheddar, Swiss, or your favorite variety)

Instructions:

1. Place crackers on a plate.

2. Top each cracker with a slice of cheese.

3. Enjoy as is or melt cheese in the microwave for a warm snack.

Nutrition Information:

- Calories: 160
- Protein: 8g
- Carbohydrates: 15g
- Fat: 8g
- Fiber: 3g
- Sugar: 1g
- Portion Size: 4 crackers and 1 slice of cheese

Edamame with Sea Salt

Ingredients:

- 1 cup edamame (fresh or frozen)
- Sea salt to taste

Instructions:

1. Cook edamame according to package instructions.

2. Sprinkle with sea salt.

3. Serve warm or chilled.

Nutrition Information:

- Calories: 120
- Protein: 11g
- Carbohydrates: 9g
- Fat: 5g
- Fiber: 4g
- Sugar: 2g
- Portion Size: 1 cup edamame

Apple Slices with Almond Butter

Ingredients:

- 1 apple, sliced
- 2 tablespoons almond butter

Instructions:

1. Slice the apple into wedges.
2. Spread almond butter on each apple slice.
3. Enjoy as a satisfying and crunchy snack.

Nutrition Information:

- Calories: 180
- Protein: 4g
- Carbohydrates: 20g
- Fat: 10g
- Fiber: 5g
- Sugar: 15g
- Portion Size: 1 apple and 2 tablespoons almond butter

Veggie Sushi Rolls

Ingredients:

- Nori seaweed sheets
- Cooked sushi rice
- Assorted vegetables (cucumber, avocado, carrot, bell pepper)
- Soy sauce and wasabi for dipping (optional)

Instructions:

1. Place a sheet of nori on a bamboo sushi mat.

2. Spread a layer of sushi rice on the nori, leaving a border at the top.

3. Arrange sliced vegetables in the center of the rice.

4. Roll up the sushi tightly using the bamboo mat.

5. Slice into pieces and serve with soy sauce and wasabi if desired.

Nutrition Information:

- Calories: 160

- Protein: 4g

- Carbohydrates: 30g

- Fat: 2g

- Fiber: 6g

- Sugar: 2g

- Portion Size: 6 pieces of sushi

Deviled Eggs with Avocado

Ingredients:

- 6 hard-boiled eggs, peeled and halved

- 1 ripe avocado

- 1 tablespoon Greek yogurt

- 1 teaspoon Dijon mustard

- Salt and pepper to taste

- Paprika for garnish

Instructions:

1. Remove egg yolks and place them in a bowl.

2. Mash the egg yolks with avocado, Greek yogurt, mustard, salt, and pepper until smooth.

3. Spoon the mixture back into the egg whites.

4. Sprinkle with paprika for garnish.

Nutrition Information:

- Calories: 130

- Protein: 8g

- Carbohydrates: 4g

- Fat: 9g

- Fiber: 3g

- Sugar: 1g

- Portion Size: 3 deviled egg halves

Kale Chips with Parmesan

Ingredients:

- 1 bunch kale, washed and dried
- 1 tablespoon olive oil
- 2 tablespoons grated Parmesan cheese
- Salt and pepper to taste

Instructions:

1. Preheat oven to 350°F (175°C).
2. Remove the stems from the kale leaves and tear into bite-sized pieces.
3. In a bowl, toss kale with olive oil, Parmesan cheese, salt, and pepper.
4. Spread kale in a single layer on a baking sheet lined with parchment paper.
5. Bake for 10-15 minutes until crispy.
6. Let cool before serving.

Nutrition Information:

- Calories: 100
- Protein: 5g

- Carbohydrates: 8g

- Fat: 6g

- Fiber: 3g

- Sugar: 1g

- Portion Size: 1 cup kale chips

Fruit Salad Skewers

Ingredients:

- Assorted fruits (strawberries, grapes, melon, pineapple)
- Wooden skewers

Instructions:

1. Wash and chop fruits into bite-sized pieces.
2. Thread fruits onto skewers in an attractive pattern.
3. Serve immediately or refrigerate until ready to eat.

Nutrition Information:

- Calories: 80

- Protein: 1g

- Carbohydrates: 20g

- Fat: 0g

- Fiber: 3g

- Sugar: 15g

- Portion Size: 1 skewer

Stuffed Mini Bell Peppers

Ingredients:

- Mini bell peppers

- Hummus or cream cheese

- Cherry tomatoes, sliced

- Cucumber, diced

- Fresh herbs (parsley, chives)

Instructions:

1. Cut the tops off mini bell peppers and remove seeds.

2. Fill each pepper with hummus or cream cheese.

3. Top with sliced cherry tomatoes, diced cucumber, and fresh herbs.

4. Serve chilled or at room temperature.

Nutrition Information:

- Calories: 70
- Protein: 2g
- Carbohydrates: 10g
- Fat: 3g
- Fiber: 2g
- Sugar: 5g
- Portion Size: 2 stuffed mini peppers

Cucumber and Tomato Salad

Ingredients:

- 2 cucumbers, sliced
- 2 tomatoes, diced
- 1/4 red onion, thinly sliced
- 2 tablespoons olive oil
- 1 tablespoon balsamic vinegar
- Salt and pepper to taste
- Fresh basil leaves for garnish

Instructions:

1. In a large bowl, combine cucumber slices, diced tomatoes, and sliced red onion.
2. Drizzle with olive oil and balsamic vinegar.
3. Season with salt and pepper, toss to coat.
4. Garnish with fresh basil leaves before serving.

Nutrition Information:

-   Calories: 90
-   Protein: 2g
-   Carbohydrates: 10g
-   Fat: 6g
-   Fiber: 3g
-   Sugar: 5g
-   Portion Size: 1 cup salad

Roasted Chickpeas with Herbs

Ingredients:

-   1 can chickpeas, drained and rinsed
-   1 tablespoon olive oil
-   1 teaspoon garlic powder

- 1 teaspoon dried herbs (rosemary, thyme, oregano)
- Salt and pepper to taste

Instructions:

1. Preheat oven to 400°F (200°C).
2. Pat chickpeas dry with a paper towel and remove any loose skins.
3. In a bowl, toss chickpeas with olive oil, garlic powder, dried herbs, salt, and pepper.
4. Spread chickpeas in a single layer on a baking sheet lined with parchment paper.
5. Roast for 25-30 minutes until crispy, shaking the pan halfway through.
6. Let cool before serving.

Nutrition Information:

- Calories: 150
- Protein: 6g
- Carbohydrates: 20g
- Fat: 5g
- Fiber: 6g
- Sugar: 3g
- Portion Size: 1/2 cup roasted chickpeas

Chapter 6: Desserts

This chapter presents a collection of delightful desserts designed with your well-being in mind. From fruity delights to rich chocolatey treats, these recipes offer a balance of flavor and nutrition, perfect for satisfying your sweet tooth without guilt.

Mixed Berry Crisp with Oat Topping

Ingredients:

- 2 cups mixed berries (strawberries, blueberries, raspberries)
- 1/4 cup rolled oats
- 2 tablespoons almond flour
- 1 tablespoon honey or maple syrup
- 1 tablespoon melted coconut oil
- Pinch of cinnamon

Instructions:

1. Preheat oven to 350°F (175°C).

2. In a mixing bowl, combine mixed berries with honey or maple syrup.

3. In a separate bowl, mix rolled oats, almond flour, melted coconut oil, and cinnamon until crumbly.

4. Spread the berry mixture evenly in a baking dish and top with the oat mixture.

5. Bake for 25-30 minutes or until the topping is golden brown and the berries are bubbling.

6. Serve warm, optionally with a scoop of Greek yogurt or a dollop of whipped cream.

Nutrition Information (per serving):

- Calories: 180
- Protein: 3g
- Carbohydrates: 25g
- Fat: 8g
- Fiber: 5g
- Sugar: 15g
- Portion size: 1/6 of the recipe

Dark Chocolate Covered Strawberries

Ingredients:

- 1 cup dark chocolate chips
- 12 large strawberries, rinsed and dried

Instructions:

1. Melt the dark chocolate chips in a microwave-safe bowl in 30-second intervals, stirring in between, until smooth.
2. Dip each strawberry into the melted chocolate, allowing any excess to drip off.
3. Place the dipped strawberries on a parchment-lined baking sheet.
4. Refrigerate for 30 minutes or until the chocolate is set.
5. Enjoy as a guilt-free indulgence!

Nutrition Information (per serving, 2 strawberries):

- Calories: 120
- Protein: 2g

- Carbohydrates: 15g

- Fat: 8g

- Fiber: 3g

- Sugar: 10g

- Portion size: 2 strawberries

Greek Yogurt Popsicles with Fruit

Ingredients:

- 1 cup Greek yogurt

- 1 cup mixed fruit (such as chopped strawberries, blueberries, and mango)

- 2 tablespoons honey or maple syrup

Instructions:

1. In a bowl, mix Greek yogurt with honey or maple syrup until well combined.

2. Layer the yogurt mixture and mixed fruit in popsicle molds.

3. Insert popsicle sticks and freeze for at least 4 hours or until solid.

4. Run warm water over the molds to release the popsicles before serving.

Nutrition Information (per serving, 1 popsicle):

- Calories: 80
- Protein: 4g
- Carbohydrates: 15g
- Fat: 0g
- Fiber: 1g
- Sugar: 12g
- Portion size: 1 popsicle

Baked Apples with Cinnamon

Ingredients:

- 2 large apples, cored and halved
- 1 tablespoon honey or maple syrup
- 1 teaspoon ground cinnamon
- 2 tablespoons chopped nuts (optional)

Instructions:

1. Preheat oven to 375°F (190°C).

2. Place apple halves cut side up in a baking dish.

3. Drizzle honey or maple syrup over the apples and sprinkle with cinnamon.

4. Bake for 20-25 minutes or until apples are tender.

5. Serve warm, optionally topped with chopped nuts for added crunch.

Nutrition Information (per serving, 1 apple half):

- Calories: 80
- Protein: 1g
- Carbohydrates: 20g
- Fat: 0g
- Fiber: 4g
- Sugar: 15g
- Portion size: 1 apple half

Chia Seed Pudding with Mango

Ingredients:

- 1/4 cup chia seeds
- 1 cup unsweetened almond milk
- 1 tablespoon honey or maple syrup

- 1/2 teaspoon vanilla extract
- 1 ripe mango, diced

Instructions:

1. In a bowl, mix chia seeds, almond milk, honey or maple syrup, and vanilla extract. Stir well.
2. Let the mixture sit for 5 minutes, then stir again to break up any clumps.
3. Cover and refrigerate for at least 2 hours or overnight until thickened.
4. Serve chilled, topped with diced mango.

Nutrition Information (per serving):

- Calories: 150
- Protein: 4g
- Carbohydrates: 20g
- Fat: 6g
- Fiber: 10g
- Sugar: 10g
- Portion size: 1/2 cup

Banana Ice Cream with Almond Butter

Ingredients:

- 2 ripe bananas, sliced and frozen
- 2 tablespoons almond butter
- Optional toppings: chopped nuts, dark chocolate chips

Instructions:

1. Place frozen banana slices in a blender or food processor.
2. Blend until smooth and creamy, scraping down the sides as needed.
3. Add almond butter and blend until fully incorporated.
4. Serve immediately as soft-serve ice cream or transfer to a container and freeze for a firmer texture.
5. Sprinkle with chopped nuts or dark chocolate chips before serving, if desired.

Nutrition Information (per serving):

- Calories: 200
- Protein: 4g
- Carbohydrates: 30g
- Fat: 8g
- Fiber: 5g
- Sugar: 15g
- Portion size: 1/2 cup

Pumpkin Spice Muffins

Ingredients:

- 1 1/2 cups almond flour
- 1/2 cup canned pumpkin puree
- 1/4 cup honey or maple syrup
- 2 eggs
- 1 teaspoon vanilla extract
- 1 teaspoon pumpkin pie spice
- 1/2 teaspoon baking powder
- Pinch of salt

Instructions:

1. Preheat oven to 350°F (175°C) and line a muffin tin with paper liners.

2. In a mixing bowl, whisk together almond flour, pumpkin puree, honey or maple syrup, eggs, vanilla extract, pumpkin pie spice, baking powder, and salt until well combined.

3. Divide the batter evenly among the muffin cups.

4. Bake for 20-25 minutes or until a toothpick inserted into the center comes out clean.

5. Allow muffins to cool in the tin for 5 minutes, then transfer to a wire rack to cool completely.

Nutrition Information (per muffin):

- Calories: 150
- Protein: 6g
- Carbohydrates: 15g
- Fat: 8g
- Fiber: 3g
- Sugar: 10g
- Portion size: 1 muffin

Avocado Chocolate Mousse

Ingredients:

- 2 ripe avocados
- 1/4 cup unsweetened cocoa powder
- 1/4 cup honey or maple syrup
- 1 teaspoon vanilla extract
- Pinch of salt
- Optional toppings: fresh berries, shaved dark chocolate

Instructions:

1. Scoop the flesh of the avocados into a blender or food processor.
2. Add cocoa powder, honey or maple syrup, vanilla extract, and salt.
3. Blend until smooth and creamy, scraping down the sides as needed.
4. Divide the mousse into serving dishes and refrigerate for at least 30 minutes to chill.
5. Serve topped with fresh berries or shaved dark chocolate, if desired.

Nutrition Information (per serving):

- Calories: 200
- Protein: 3g
- Carbohydrates: 20g
- Fat: 15g
- Fiber: 7g
- Sugar: 10g
- Portion size: 1/2 cup

Lemon Blueberry Bars

Ingredients:

- 1 cup almond flour
- 1/4 cup coconut flour
- 1/4 cup honey or maple syrup
- 1/4 cup melted coconut oil
- Zest and juice of 1 lemon
- 1 cup fresh blueberries
- Pinch of salt

Instructions:

1. Preheat oven to 350°F (175°C) and line an 8x8-inch baking dish with parchment paper.
2. In a mixing bowl, combine almond flour, coconut flour, honey or maple syrup, melted coconut oil, lemon zest, and salt until a dough forms.
3. Press the dough evenly into the bottom of the prepared baking dish.
4. Scatter blueberries over the dough and gently press them in.
5. Bake for 20-25 minutes or until the edges are golden brown.
6. Let cool completely before slicing into bars.

Nutrition Information (per bar):

- Calories: 120
- Protein: 2g
- Carbohydrates: 15g
- Fat: 6g
- Fiber: 3g
- Sugar: 8g
- Portion size: 1 bar

Coconut Macaroons

Ingredients:

- 2 cups shredded coconut (unsweetened)
- 1/2 cup coconut flour
- 1/4 cup honey or maple syrup
- 1/4 cup melted coconut oil
- 2 eggs
- 1 teaspoon vanilla extract
- Pinch of salt

Instructions:

1. Preheat oven to 325°F (160°C) and line a baking sheet with parchment paper.
2. In a large bowl, combine shredded coconut, coconut flour, honey or maple syrup, melted coconut oil, eggs, vanilla extract, and salt. Mix well until a sticky dough forms.
3. Use a tablespoon to scoop out portions of the dough and shape into small mounds.
4. Place the mounds on the prepared baking sheet, spacing them apart.
5. Bake for 15-18 minutes or until golden brown.

6. Let the macaroons cool on the baking sheet for 5 minutes, then transfer to a wire rack to cool completely.

Nutrition Information (per macaroon):

- Calories: 100
- Protein: 2g
- Carbohydrates: 10g
- Fat: 7g
- Fiber: 2g
- Sugar: 6g
- Portion size: 1 macaroon

Almond Flour Brownies

Ingredients:

- 1 cup almond flour
- 1/4 cup cocoa powder
- 1/4 cup honey or maple syrup
- 1/4 cup melted coconut oil
- 2 eggs
- 1 teaspoon vanilla extract

- 1/4 teaspoon baking soda
- Pinch of salt

Instructions:

1. Preheat oven to 350°F (175°C) and line an 8x8-inch baking dish with parchment paper.
2. In a mixing bowl, combine almond flour, cocoa powder, honey or maple syrup, melted coconut oil, eggs, vanilla extract, baking soda, and salt. Mix until well combined.
3. Pour the batter into the prepared baking dish and spread it evenly.
4. Bake for 20-25 minutes or until a toothpick inserted into the center comes out clean.
5. Let the brownies cool in the pan for 10 minutes, then transfer to a wire rack to cool completely before slicing.

Nutrition Information (per brownie):

- Calories: 120
- Protein: 3g
- Carbohydrates: 10g

- Fat: 8g

- Fiber: 2g

- Sugar: 6g

- Portion size: 1 brownie

Strawberry Frozen Yogurt Bark

Ingredients:

- 2 cups Greek yogurt

- 1 cup sliced strawberries

- 2 tablespoons honey or maple syrup

- 1/4 cup chopped nuts (optional)

Instructions:

1. Line a baking sheet with parchment paper.

2. Spread Greek yogurt evenly on the parchment paper, about 1/4 inch thick.

3. Arrange sliced strawberries on top of the yogurt.

4. Drizzle honey or maple syrup over the strawberries.

5. Sprinkle chopped nuts evenly over the top, if desired.

6. Place the baking sheet in the freezer for at least 3 hours or until the yogurt bark is frozen solid.

7. Once frozen, break the bark into pieces and serve immediately.

Nutrition Information (per serving, 1/6 of the bark):

- Calories: 100
- Protein: 6g
- Carbohydrates: 10g
- Fat: 4g
- Fiber: 1g
- Sugar: 8g
- Portion size: 1/6 of the bark

Pineapple Sorbet

Ingredients:

- 2 cups frozen pineapple chunks
- 1/4 cup coconut water or pineapple juice
- 2 tablespoons honey or maple syrup
- Juice of 1 lime

Instructions:

1. In a blender or food processor, combine frozen pineapple chunks, coconut water or pineapple juice, honey or maple syrup, and lime juice.

2. Blend until smooth and creamy, scraping down the sides as needed.

3. If the mixture is too thick, add more liquid a little at a time until desired consistency is reached.

4. Transfer the sorbet to a container and freeze for 1-2 hours to firm up.

5. Serve in bowls or scoops, garnished with fresh mint leaves if desired.

Nutrition Information (per serving, 1/2 cup):

- Calories: 90
- Protein: 1g
- Carbohydrates: 25g
- Fat: 0g
- Fiber: 2g
- Sugar: 20g
- Portion size: 1/2 cup

Carrot Cake Bites

Ingredients:

- 1 cup shredded carrots
- 1/2 cup dates, pitted
- 1/2 cup rolled oats
- 1/4 cup shredded coconut (unsweetened)
- 1/4 cup chopped walnuts
- 1 teaspoon cinnamon
- 1/4 teaspoon nutmeg
- Pinch of salt

Instructions:

1. In a food processor, combine shredded carrots, dates, rolled oats, shredded coconut, chopped walnuts, cinnamon, nutmeg, and salt.
2. Pulse until the mixture comes together and forms a sticky dough.
3. Scoop out tablespoon-sized portions of the dough and roll into balls.
4. Place the carrot cake bites on a plate or baking sheet lined with parchment paper.

5. Refrigerate for at least 30 minutes to firm up before serving.

Nutrition Information (per bite):

- Calories: 80
- Protein: 2g
- Carbohydrates: 15g
- Fat: 3g
- Fiber: 2g
- Sugar: 10g
- Portion size: 1 bite

Berry Parfait with Greek Yogurt

Ingredients:

- 1 cup Greek yogurt
- 1/2 cup mixed berries (strawberries, blueberries, raspberries)
- 2 tablespoons granola
- 1 tablespoon honey or maple syrup

Instructions:

1. In a serving glass or bowl, layer Greek yogurt, mixed berries, and granola.

2. Drizzle honey or maple syrup over the top.

3. Repeat the layers until the glass or bowl is filled.

4. Serve immediately as a nutritious and delicious dessert or snack option.

Nutrition Information (per serving):

- Calories: 150

- Protein: 10g

- Carbohydrates: 20g

- Fat: 4g

- Fiber: 3g

- Sugar: 12g

- Portion size: 1 serving

Chapter 7: Smoothies

These refreshing blends are not only delicious but also packed with nutrients to support your health journey. Whether you're looking for a quick breakfast option, a post-workout refuel, or a satisfying snack, these smoothie recipes have got you covered.

Green Detox Smoothie

Ingredients:

- 1 cup spinach
- 1/2 cucumber, peeled and chopped
- 1/2 green apple, cored and chopped
- 1/2 lemon, juiced
- 1/2 cup coconut water
- Ice cubes, as desired

Instructions:

1. Place all ingredients in a blender.
2. Blend until smooth.

3. Pour into a glass and enjoy!

Nutrition Information (per serving):

- Calories: 80
- Protein: 2g
- Carbohydrates: 18g
- Fat: 0g
- Fiber: 4g
- Sugar: 10g
- Portion size: 1 serving

Berry Blast Smoothie

Ingredients:

- 1/2 cup mixed berries (strawberries, blueberries, raspberries)
- 1/2 banana, frozen
- 1/2 cup Greek yogurt
- 1/2 cup almond milk
- 1 tablespoon honey (optional)

Instructions:

1. Combine all ingredients in a blender.
2. Blend until smooth and creamy.
3. Pour into a glass and enjoy!

Nutrition Information (per serving):

- Calories: 150
- Protein: 6g
- Carbohydrates: 30g
- Fat: 1g
- Fiber: 5g
- Sugar: 22g
- Portion size: 1 serving

Tropical Paradise Smoothie

Ingredients:

- 1/2 cup pineapple chunks
- 1/2 cup mango chunks
- 1/2 banana, frozen
- 1/2 cup coconut milk
- Ice cubes, as desired

Instructions:

1. Add all ingredients to a blender.

2. Blend until smooth and creamy.

3. Pour into a glass and enjoy the taste of the tropics!

Nutrition Information (per serving):

- Calories: 200

- Protein: 3g

- Carbohydrates: 40g

- Fat: 5g

- Fiber: 5g

- Sugar: 30g

- Portion size: 1 serving

Chocolate Banana Protein Smoothie

Ingredients:

- 1 scoop chocolate protein powder

- 1/2 banana, frozen

- 1 tablespoon almond butter

- 1 cup almond milk

- Ice cubes, as desired

Instructions:

1. Place all ingredients in a blender.

2. Blend until smooth and creamy.

3. Pour into a glass and enjoy this indulgent yet nutritious treat!

Nutrition Information (per serving):

- Calories: 280
- Protein: 20g
- Carbohydrates: 25g
- Fat: 10g
- Fiber: 5g
- Sugar: 10g
- Portion size: 1 serving

Mango Tango Smoothie

Ingredients:

- 1 cup mango chunks
- 1/2 cup orange juice
- 1/2 cup Greek yogurt
- 1 tablespoon honey (optional)

- Ice cubes, as desired

Instructions:

1. Combine all ingredients in a blender.

2. Blend until smooth and creamy.

3. Pour into a glass and savor the tropical flavors!

Nutrition Information (per serving):

- Calories: 180

- Protein: 7g

- Carbohydrates: 35g

- Fat: 1g

- Fiber: 3g

- Sugar: 30g

- Portion size: 1 serving

Peanut Butter and Banana Smoothie

Ingredients:

- 1/2 banana, frozen

- 1 tablespoon peanut butter

- 1/2 cup Greek yogurt

- 1/2 cup almond milk

- Ice cubes, as desired

Instructions:

1. Add all ingredients to a blender.

2. Blend until smooth and creamy.

3. Pour into a glass and enjoy the classic combination of peanut butter and banana!

Nutrition Information (per serving):

- Calories: 250

- Protein: 15g

- Carbohydrates: 25g

- Fat: 10g

- Fiber: 3g

- Sugar: 15g

- Portion size: 1 serving

Spinach and Pineapple Smoothie

Ingredients:

- 1 cup spinach

- 1/2 cup pineapple chunks
- 1/2 banana, frozen
- 1/2 cup coconut water
- Ice cubes, as desired

Instructions:

1. Place all ingredients in a blender.
2. Blend until smooth and creamy.
3. Pour into a glass and enjoy this refreshing green smoothie!

Nutrition Information (per serving):

- Calories: 120
- Protein: 3g
- Carbohydrates: 25g
- Fat: 1g
- Fiber: 4g
- Sugar: 15g
- Portion size: 1 serving

Peach and Almond Smoothie

Ingredients:

- 1 cup sliced peaches
- 1/4 cup almonds
- 1/2 cup Greek yogurt
- 1/2 cup almond milk
- Ice cubes, as desired

Instructions:

1. Combine all ingredients in a blender.
2. Blend until smooth and creamy.
3. Pour into a glass and enjoy the delightful combination of peach and almond flavors!

Nutrition Information (per serving):

- Calories: 220
- Protein: 10g
- Carbohydrates: 30g
- Fat: 8g
- Fiber: 5g
- Sugar: 20g
- Portion size: 1 serving

Kale and Berry Smoothie

Ingredients:

- 1 cup kale leaves, stems removed
- 1/2 cup mixed berries (strawberries, blueberries, raspberries)
- 1/2 banana, frozen
- 1/2 cup almond milk
- Ice cubes, as desired

Instructions:

1. Add all ingredients to a blender.
2. Blend until smooth and creamy.
3. Pour into a glass and enjoy the nutritious boost of kale and berries!

Nutrition Information (per serving):

- Calories: 150
- Protein: 5g
- Carbohydrates: 30g
- Fat: 2g
- Fiber: 6g

- Sugar: 18g
- Portion size: 1 serving

Orange Creamsicle Smoothie

Ingredients:

- 1/2 cup orange juice
- 1/2 cup Greek yogurt
- 1/2 banana, frozen
- 1/2 teaspoon vanilla extract
- Ice cubes, as desired

Instructions:

1. Combine all ingredients in a blender.
2. Blend until smooth and creamy.
3. Pour into a glass and enjoy the nostalgic taste of an orange creamsicle!

Nutrition Information (per serving):

- Calories: 160
- Protein: 8g
- Carbohydrates: 30g

- Fat: 1g
- Fiber: 2g
- Sugar: 20g
- Portion size: 1 serving

Beet and Berry Smoothie

Ingredients:

- 1/2 cup cooked beets, chopped
- 1/2 cup mixed berries (strawberries, blueberries, raspberries)
- 1/2 cup Greek yogurt
- 1/2 cup almond milk
- Ice cubes, as desired

Instructions:

1. Place all ingredients in a blender.
2. Blend until smooth and creamy.
3. Pour into a glass and enjoy the vibrant color and flavor of this beet and berry smoothie!

Nutrition Information (per serving):

- Calories: 180
- Protein: 7g
- Carbohydrates: 30g
- Fat: 3g
- Fiber: 5g
- Sugar: 20g
- Portion size: 1 serving

Cucumber Mint Smoothie

Ingredients:

- 1/2 cucumber, peeled and chopped
- 1/4 cup fresh mint leaves
- 1/2 cup Greek yogurt
- 1/2 cup coconut water
- Ice cubes, as desired

Instructions:

1. Add all ingredients to a blender.
2. Blend until smooth and refreshing.

3. Pour into a glass and enjoy the cooling sensation of cucumber and mint!

Nutrition Information (per serving):

- Calories: 90
- Protein: 6g
- Carbohydrates: 15g
- Fat: 1g
- Fiber: 2g
- Sugar: 10g
- Portion size: 1 serving

Blueberry Oatmeal Smoothie

Ingredients:

- 1/2 cup blueberries
- 1/4 cup rolled oats
- 1/2 banana, frozen
- 1/2 cup Greek yogurt
- 1/2 cup almond milk
- Ice cubes, as desired

Instructions:

1. Combine all ingredients in a blender.
2. Blend until smooth and creamy.
3. Pour into a glass and enjoy the satisfying texture and flavor of this blueberry oatmeal smoothie!

Nutrition Information (per serving):

- Calories: 220
- Protein: 12g
- Carbohydrates: 35g
- Fat: 4g
- Fiber: 6g
- Sugar: 18g
- Portion size: 1 serving

Carrot Cake Smoothie

Ingredients:

- 1/2 cup shredded carrots
- 1/4 cup rolled oats
- 1/2 banana, frozen
- 1/2 teaspoon cinnamon

- 1 tablespoon honey (optional)
- 1/2 cup almond milk
- Ice cubes, as desired

Instructions:

1. Place all ingredients in a blender.
2. Blend until smooth and creamy.
3. Pour into a glass and enjoy the taste of carrot cake in a healthy smoothie form!

Nutrition Information (per serving):

- Calories: 230
- Protein: 8g
- Carbohydrates: 40g
- Fat: 4g
- Fiber: 7g
- Sugar: 18g
- Portion size: 1 serving

Avocado Kale Smoothie

Ingredients:

- 1/2 avocado
- 1 cup kale leaves, stems removed
- 1/2 cup pineapple chunks
- 1/2 cup Greek yogurt
- 1/2 cup coconut water
- Ice cubes, as desired

Instructions:

1. Add all ingredients to a blender.
2. Blend until smooth and creamy.
3. Pour into a glass and enjoy the creamy texture and nutritious benefits of this avocado kale smoothie!

Nutrition Information (per serving):

- Calories: 220
- Protein: 9g
- Carbohydrates: 25g
- Fat: 10g
- Fiber: 7g
- Sugar: 15g
- Portion size: 1 serving

CONCLUSION

As we close the pages of the "Stroke and Diabetes Diet Cookbook," we embark on a journey that goes far beyond mere recipes. This book is a testament to the power of nutrition in not just managing, but thriving with conditions like stroke and diabetes. Through careful curation of balanced meals, thoughtful consideration of ingredients, and creative culinary techniques, we've crafted a collection that nourishes both body and soul.

But this cookbook is more than just a collection of recipes—it's a roadmap to a healthier, more vibrant life. It's a reminder that even in the face of health challenges, we hold the reins of our well-being. Each dish represents a choice, a step towards wellness, and a commitment to self-care.

As you savor the flavors and textures of these dishes, may you also savor the journey towards better health. Celebrate every meal enjoyed mindfully, every vegetable chopped with intention, and every bite savored with gratitude.

But our journey doesn't end here. Let this cookbook be a starting point, a foundation upon which to build a lifetime of healthy eating habits. Explore, experiment, and adapt these recipes to suit your taste preferences and dietary needs. And remember, the kitchen is your sanctuary, a place where you can nourish not just your body, but your spirit as well.

As you continue on your path to wellness, know that you're not alone. Lean on the support of loved ones, seek guidance from healthcare professionals, and find inspiration in the vibrant community of individuals striving for better health alongside you.

So here's to you, to your health, and to the countless delicious meals yet to be enjoyed. May this cookbook be a trusted companion on your journey towards a life filled with vitality, joy, and delicious, nourishing food.

www.ingramcontent.com/pod-product-compliance
Lightning Source LLC
Chambersburg PA
CBHW071007250726
48653CB00005B/1544